T0132386

POSTURE, SIMPLY POSTURE, CORRECT SIMPLY

Polixeni Katsaros, PT, DPT

Archway Publishing books may be ordered through booksellers or by contacting:

Archway Publishing
1663 Liberty Drive
Bloomington, IN 47403
www.archwaypublishing.com
1 (888) 242-5904

ISBN: 978-1-4808-8218-8 (sc)
ISBN: 978-1-4808-8219-5 (hc)
ISBN: 978-1-4808-8217-1 (e)

Print information available on the last page.

Archway Publishing rev. date: 09/03/2019

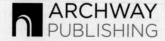

Preface

Unless we are in water or outer space, gravity affects all our bodies; it is a constant force upon us.

This book is about Posture, suitable for all ages.

Since we live on earth and we experience gravity, we need to understand how to align ourselves when gravity's forces are upon us, so we are not stressing the muscles.

To the memory of Mom and Baba
To all my patients, you know who you are

Introduction

This is a guide for preventing backaches. If you understand your body's anatomy and how it works, then you have the ability to practice posture correction.

In this book, I educate you about the importance of posture and the ability to correct it, as Slouch and Correct do.

I have been dedicated to the practice of physical therapy for more than thirty years and focused my practice on teaching people of all ages postural correction through functional movement.

Everything we do throughout our lives affects our spines, and it is inevitable that we put repeated stress on our backs.

My message is that *you* can reverse the effects of stress on your back. It is my intention to reach as many people as possible to teach the basic tools needed for a healthy back—quite simply, correct posture.

First, it is important to know a few basics of anatomy: pelvis, spine, discs, nerves, ligaments, and muscles.

Our bodies are strong as long as we align our spine, sounds easy, right? But the fact is we don't pay attention to our spine until our muscles begin to ache and hurt.

Muscles are designed to make us move, and we don't have to think about moving since our nervous system connects to all our muscles automatically. However, life places us in situations where we demand more from our muscles than responding to the forces of gravity.

Our bodies' way of letting us know that our spine alignment is off or that our muscles are being asked to do more than they can handle is by feeling achy back pain.

The problem is that we often ignore for too long the important messages our bodies are telling each of us.

So who is responsible? You are! We all are responsible for setting the example for our children and our loved ones all around us.

In this book you will meet the following characters:

- MegaMuscle,
- SlinkySpine,
- BravoPelvis,
- Gravity

We see MegaMuscle's emotions displayed with a happy face when BravoPelvis and SlinkySpine are aligned and a sad face when BravoPelvis and SlinkySpine are not aligned.

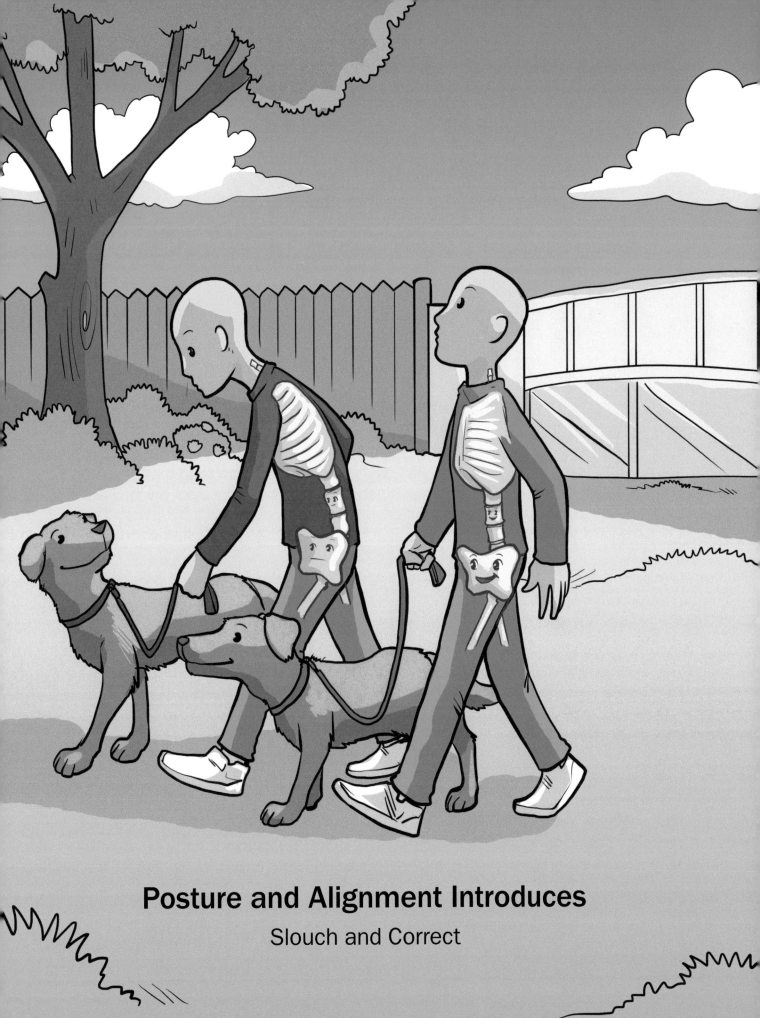

Posture and Alignment Introduces

Slouch and Correct

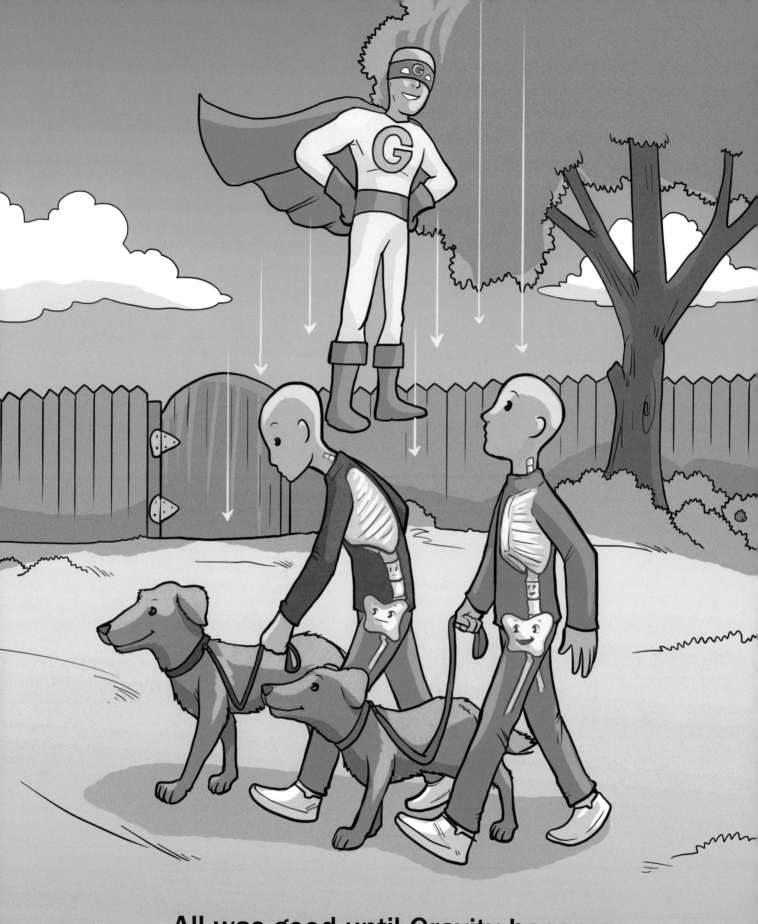

All was good until Gravity became
present and permanent in effect.

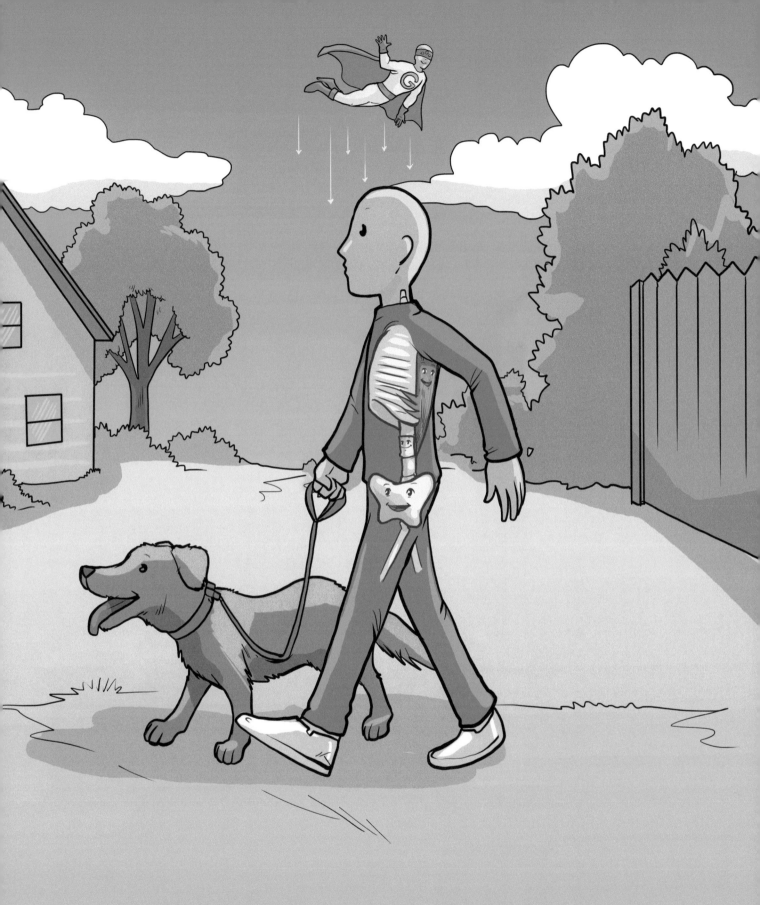

Better understand how the straighter
you stand changes Gravity's effect.

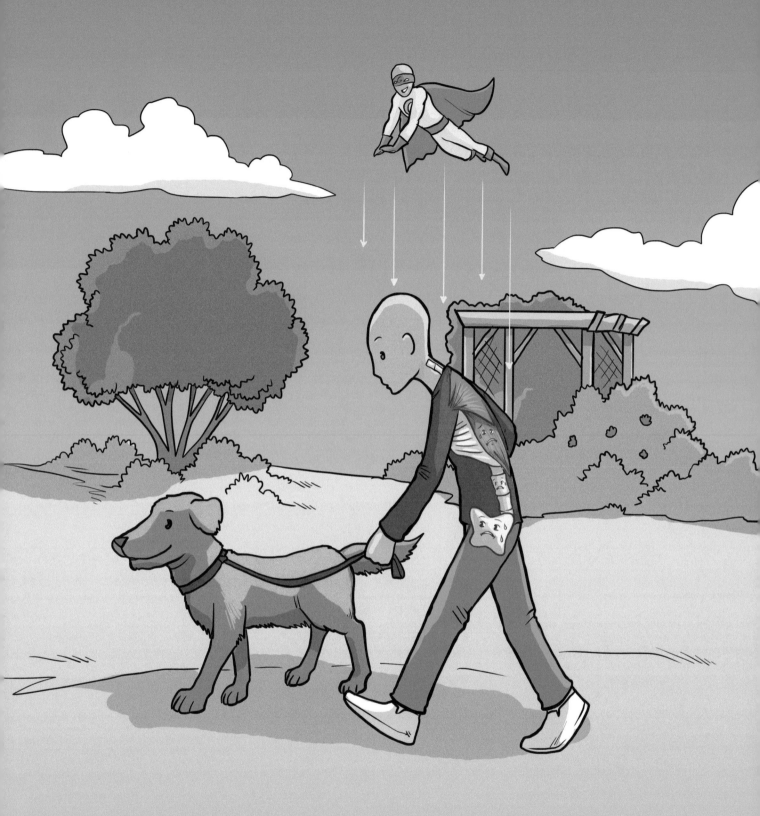

So Slouch is feeling muscle pain later that day.

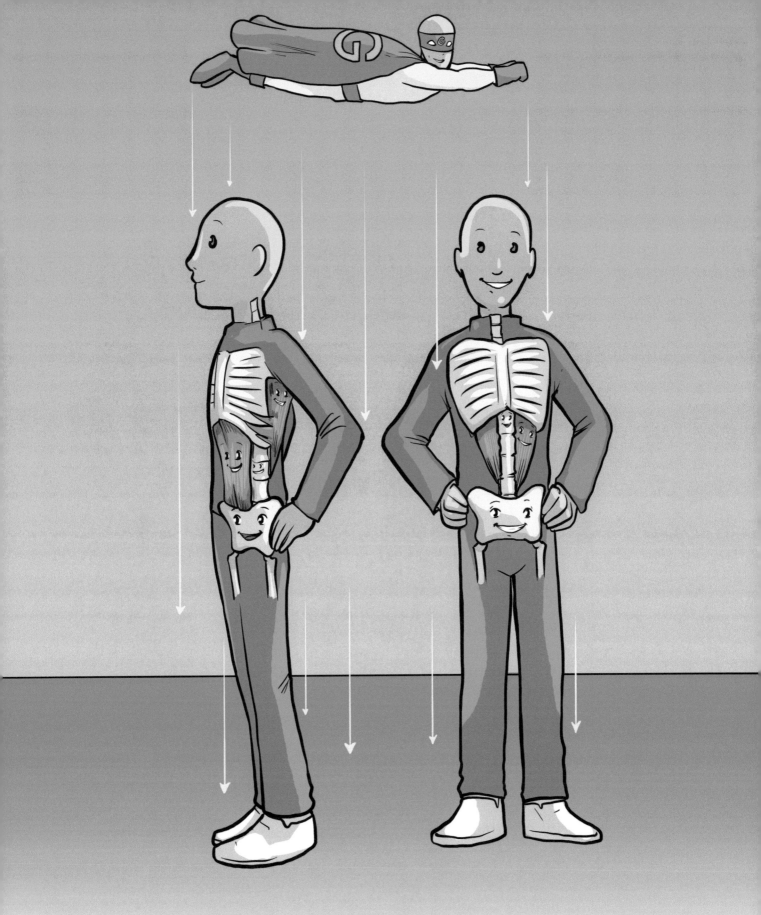

Meanwhile, Correct understands Gravity's effect.

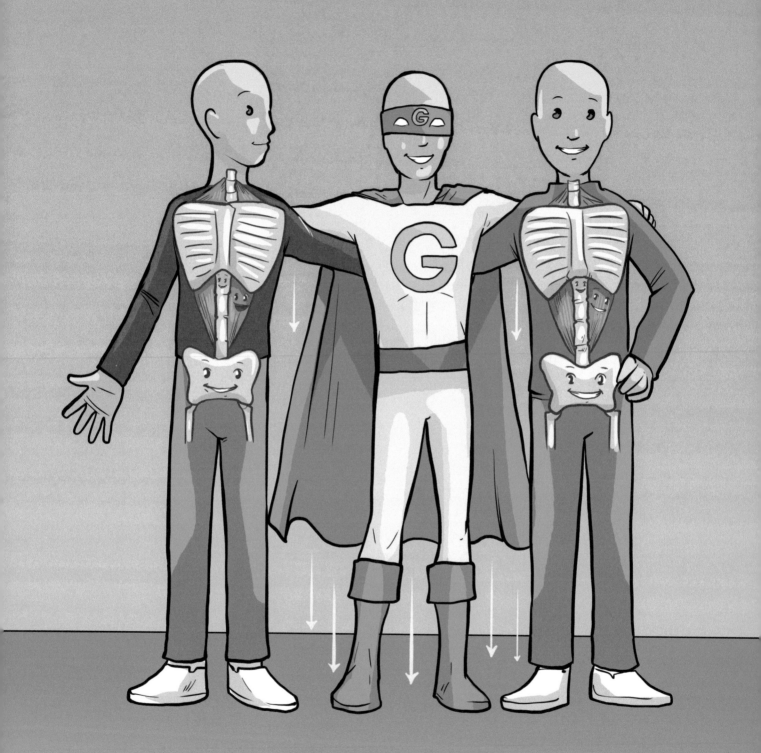

Then Slouch and Correct grew to understand what
and why to align for simple posture simply.

AFTERWORD

When should you perform correct posture? Anytime you think about it—during a TV commercial, waiting at a traffic light, sitting in a meeting, waiting for a teacher or friend, or before and after car rides.

Many times throughout a given day, correct posture is not only possible but *simple.*

What if every time you bent forward, you bent backward to counteract the stresses? Practicing correct posture is easy if you are able to move. Correct posture becomes easier when you practice posture *simply*.

Correct Posture in Sitting

- Sit on a firm surface with your hips level with or slightly higher than your knees with your feet on the floor.
- Engage your abdominal muscles to stabilize your pelvis.
- Raise your breastbone up,
- Bring your head back and chin level.
- Breathe in and out through your nose, maintaining correctly aligned posture for an entire inhale and exhale, and then relax.

Repeat the slouch correction throughout the day.

Correct Posture in Standing

- Stand with your feet shoulder-width apart
- Shift your weight forward
- Engage your abdominal muscles to stabilize your pelvis
- Raise your breastbone upward
- Bringing your head back and your chin level.
- Breathe in and out through your nose.

Acknowledgments

I want to thank my wife, Joanne; my brothers, Pantelis and Johnlee; and my sisters-in law, Deanne and Eileen, for loving me and supporting me in all I do.

I thank my nieces, Emily and Dani; my nephews, Athan, Joseph, and Tommy; and many friends and family who took the time to give me their feedback to make this book what it is. Thank you to April for editing my first draft, to Debbie for your forever energy to keep it going, and to Dottye for our late-night visits.

Printed in the United States
By Bookmasters